Black Beans and Mushroom Chili

Split Pea Soup

Pumpkin Goulash 5

Beef Rolls 6

Spinach-Mushroom-Quiche 7

Chile Verde Lasagna 8

Eggplant Sauce 9

Beef Tacos 10

Chili Slow Cooker Style 11

Chicken Enchilada Slow Cooker Style 13

Overnight Oatmeal 14

Sauerkraut Soup 15

Sausage with Celery and Chicken 16

Cabbage Rolls 17

Sweet and Sour Chicken 18

Chickpea Curry 19

Roast Turkey 20

Potato Soup 21

Vegetarian Chili 22

Spinach Sauce Slow Cooker Style 23

Vegetarian Minestrone 24

Chickpea-Squash-Lentil-Stew 25

Chickpea-Eggplant-Stew 26

Bean-Barley-Soup 27

Squash Quinoa Casserole 28

Imprint 30

Black Beans and Mushroom Chili

Ingredients:
500 g of black beans
1 tablespoon of extra virgin olive oil
25 g of mustard seeds
2 tablespoons of chili powder
1 ½ teaspoons of cumin
½ teaspoon of cardamom
2 onions, chopped
500 g of mushrooms, chopped
240 g of tomatillos, husk them and rinse and chop
60 ml of water
1400 ml of mushroom broth
180 g of tomato paste
2 tablespoons of minced garlic
150 g of pepper jack cheese (semi-hard cheese)
120 g of sour cream
25 g of cilantro
2 limes cut into wedges

Method:
1. Place the beans in a large pot with water and boil on medium to high heat for about an hour.
2. Drain and mix in the rest of the ingredients in a Dutch oven.
3. Cook on low to medium heat for about five hours.
4. Serve and enjoy, try with some sour cream and shredded cheese.

Nutritional Information:
Calories: 306 | Fat: 10 g | Carbohydrates: 40 g | Protein: 18 g

Split Pea Soup

Ingredients:

500 g of split peas
1 onion, chopped
3 carrots, chopped
3 stalks of celery, chopped
2 cloves of garlic, minced
1/8 teaspoon of pepper
1 pinch of red pepper flakes
2 liter of chicken broth

Method:

1. Chop everything up that needs to get cut and place all of the ingredients into the slow cooker.
2. Cook on high heat for about five hours, stirring every so often.
3. Serve and enjoy.

Nutritional Information:

Calories: 273 | Fat: 4 g | Carbohydrates: 44 g | Protein: 18 g

Pumpkin Goulash

Ingredients:

6 diced tomatoes
1 tablespoon of brown sugar
2 tablespoons of olive oil
1 onion, chopped
1 teaspoon of ginger
1 teaspoon of cinnamon
1 teaspoon of cumin
1 tablespoon of coriander
1 can of garbanzo beans
1.5 kg of fresh pumpkin, peeled and cut into small chunks
1 teaspoon of salt
1 teaspoon of cornstarch
60 ml of water

Method:

1. Peel and cut the pumpkin up.
2. Chop up everything else that needs to get cut up.
3. Place it all in the slow cooker.
4. Cook on high heat for about four hours.
5. Serve and enjoy.

Nutritional Information:

Calories: 330 | Fat: 8 g | Carbohydrates: 37 g | Protein: 28 g

Beef Rolls

Ingredients:

750 g beef brisket
2 onions, thinly sliced into rings
2 tbsp corn starch
2 tbsp cold water
270 g chili sauce
1 bay leaf
½ tsp dried thyme (crushed)
2 tbsp granular sugar substitute
1 garlic clove, minced
10 Italian Bread Rolls

Method:

1. Start by trimming off any excess fat from the beef. Place it in a 6 quart/6-7 liter slow cooker along with onions and bay leaf.
2. In a mixing bowl, mix the chili sauce with beer, sugar substitute, thyme, salt, pepper and garlic. Combine well and pour it over the meat.
3. Cover the cooker and cook on low heat for approximately 10-12 hours.
4. Once the beef is cooked, transfer it along with the onions onto a serving platter and cover it with a foil.
5. Next, in a medium sauce pan, pour the remaining mixture and stir it together with cornstarch and water. Cook the mixture for approximately 2 to 3 minutes or until the gravy thickens.
6. Serve the beef on the Italian rolls and top it off with the gravy.

Nutritional Information:

Calories; 325 | Fat: 8 g | Carbohydrates: 35 g | Protein: 25 g

Spinach-Mushroom-Quiche

Ingredients:

Disposable liner and non-stick cooking spray/cooking oil to grease
1 package (about 300 g) frozen chopped spinach, thawed and drained
4 slices bacon
1 tablespoon olive oil
150 g Portobello mushrooms; coarsely chopped
90 g sweet red pepper; chopped
150 g grated Swiss cheese
8 eggs
500 ml whole milk or half and half
2 tablespoons fresh chives; snipped
½ teaspoon salt
½ teaspoon black pepper
50 g biscuit mix

Method:

1. Line the slow cooker and spray liner with non-stick spray.
2. Cook bacon until crisp; drain and crumble.
3. Heat olive oil and add mushrooms and pepper. Cook until tender then add spinach and cheese.
4. Combine eggs, milk, chives, salt, and pepper and stir into spinach mixture. Add the biscuit mixture and gently fold. Pour into slow cooker and sprinkle with prepared bacon crumbs.
5. Cook in slow cooker on low for 4 to 5 hours. If using high heat cook for 2 to 2.5 hours. Cool 15 to 30 minutes before serving.

Nutritional Information:

Calories; 431 | Fat: 31 g | Carbohydrates: 66 g | Protein: 25 g

Chile Verde Lasagna

Ingredients:

500 g bulk breakfast sausage
150 g chopped sweet green pepper; finely chopped
1 jalapeno pepper; stemmed, seeded, and finely chopped
5 eggs beaten lightly
2 teaspoons vegetable oil
25 g green onions; sliced
¼ snipped cilantro or parsley
½ teaspoon salt
½ teaspoon cumin
9 corn tortillas; 6 inch/15 cm
200 g hard cheese of your choice (e.g. Monterey Jack Cheese); shredded
1x 480 g jar green salsa

Method:

1. Lightly coat the inside of the slow cooker with non-stick cooking spray.
2. Brown sausage in skillet and drain off fat. Add the sweet pepper and jalapeno pepper to skillet and cook over medium heat for 1 minute. Transfer sausage and peppers to bowl.
3. In the same pan cook eggs in hot oil just until set; stir to break up eggs. Combine eggs with sausage and peppers. Stir in green onions, cilantro, salt, and cumin.
4. Place 3 of the tortillas in the bottom of the slow cooker; it is fine if they overlap. Put half the egg and sausage mixture in the slow cooker and sprinkle with ½ cup of the cheese.
5. Pour 2/3 of the salsa over the mixture in slow cooker. Continue layering until all tortillas, sausage mixture, and salsa are in slow cooker.
6. Cover and set to low heat for 3 to 4 hours. Let stand for 15 minute before serving. Can top with sour cream and cilantro if desired.

Nutritional Information:

Calories; 429 | Fat: 29 g | Carbohydrates: 18 g | Protein: 21 g

Eggplant Sauce

Ingredients:
1 eggplant
2x 480 g cans diced tomatoes (or about 1 kg fresh chopped tomatoes)
180 g tomato paste
120 g sliced mushrooms; drained
60 ml red wine, dry
60 ml water
75 g onion, chopped
2 cloves of garlic, chopped
1½ teaspoon oregano
50 g olives, pitted
2 tablespoons fresh parsley; chopped
Black pepper
Parmesan cheese, shredded

Method:
1. Peel eggplant and cut into small cubes
2. In the slow cooker combine the eggplant, onion, canned tomatoes with juice, tomato paste, mushrooms, wine, water, garlic, and oregano.
3. Cover the slow cooker and allow it to cook on low heat for approximately 7 to 8 hours.
4. Add the olives and parsley.
5. Serve over cooked noodles and sprinkle with Parmesan cheese.

Nutritional Information:
Calories; 346 | Fat: 4 g | Carbohydrates: 65 g | Protein: 13 g

Beef Tacos

Ingredients:
1.5 kg beef; trimmed and cut into 2 inch/5 cm cubes
1 large onion; sliced thin
4 chopped cloves of garlic
1 to 3 tablespoons chopped chipotle; canned in adobo sauce
1 teaspoon oregano
2 bay leaves
Pinch of salt
400 g cabbage; thinly sliced
4 radishes, halved and thinly sliced
15 g fresh cilantro
2 tablespoons lime juice
A few Corn tortillas
Toppings: sour cream, salsa, jalapenos, shredded cheese

Method:
1. In the slow cooker toss together the beef, garlic, onion, chipotles, oregano, bay leaves, and salt. (tip: add just a bit of water to bottom to avoid sticking)
2. Cook on high for 3.5 to 4 hour or on low for 7 to 8 hours.
3. Twenty minutes before meat mixture is done wrap tortillas in foil and place in 350°F/180°C oven for 5 to 10 minutes to warm.
4. While tortillas are warming and meat is finishing up, toss together the cabbage, radishes, lime juice, and ¼ teaspoon salt.
5. Transfer the meat to a bowl and shred with a fork; save the broth. Strain the liquid into the meat and stir to combine.
6. Fill tortillas with beef and slaw; top with your choice of toppings.

Nutritional Information:
Calories; 521 | Fat: 6 g | Carbohydrates: 34 g | Protein: 57 g

Chili Slow Cooker Style

Ingredients:
500 g ground pork
500 g pork shoulder; trimmed and cut into ½ inch/1 cm cubes
300 g bell pepper; chopped
450 g chopped onion
3 minced cloves of garlic
3 tablespoons tomato paste
250 ml beer; lager style
3 tablespoons chili powder
1 tablespoon cumin
2 teaspoons oregano
¾ teaspoon black pepper
1 tomatillo, sliced
2 bay leaves
900 g plum tomatoes, chopped
450 g pinto beans, drained
220 g Mexican style tomato sauce
1 smoked ham hock
1 ½ tablespoon sugar
25 g cilantro; chopped finely
50 g green onion; chopped finely
70 g crumbled queso fresco (Mexican soft cheese)
8 lime wedges

Method:

1. Brown pork in skillet and transfer to slow cooker after draining fat.
2. Brown pork should pieces in skillet until browned and transfer to slow cooker after draining fat.
3. In skill sprayed with non-stick spray sauté onion and pepper for 8 minutes; stirring often. Add garlic and sauté 1 minute more. Add tomato paste and cook for 1 minute; stirring constantly. Stir in beer and continue cooking for 1 minute. Add onion mixture to slow cooker with meat.
4. Add chili powder, cumin, pepper, tomatillos, bay leaves, plum tomatoes, beans, tomato sauce, and ham hock. Cover and set slow cooker on high for 5 hours.
5. Remove bay leaves and ham hock; discard. Stir in sugar.
6. Ladle into serving cups or bowls; top with 1 tablespoon cilantro, cheese, green onions, and serve with a lime wedge.

Nutritional Information:

Calories; 357 | Fat: 14 g | Carbohydrates: 26 g | Protein: 28 g

Chicken Enchilada Slow Cooker Style

Ingredients:

1 teaspoon canola oil

100 g onion; chopped

60 g poblano, seeded and chopped

2 minced cloves garlic

1 ½ teaspoon chipotle chili powder

450 g diced tomatoes

240 g tomato sauce, Italian seasoned

Cooking spray or cooking oil (to grease)

280 g rotisserie chicken breast; shredded

175 g frozen; white and yellow corn

450 g black beans, drained and rinsed

5 corn and flour tortillas

240 g shredded cheddar cheese; reduced fat

Cilantro sprigs

Method:

1. Using a nonstick skillet heat on medium and add oil. Add onion, pepper, and garlic; cook until tender; about 6 minutes
2. Stir in chili powder, tomatoes, and tomato sauce. Put half the tomato mixture in a blender. Remove lid of blender and let steam escape. Place a towel over blender and blend until almost smooth and pour into a bowl. Repeat process with the other half of tomato mixture.
3. Spray slow cooker with non-stick cooking spray or grease with cooking oil. Spread 3 tablespoons of tomato mixture on bottom of slow cooker. Mix the remainder of tomato mixture with chicken, corn, and beans.
4. Place one tortilla on the tomato mixture in slow cooker. Cover with half of the chicken mixture. Sprinkle with cheese; about ¼ of the total amount. Top with another tortilla and repeat process until all tortillas and chicken mixture are in slow cooker.
5. Cook on low setting for 2 hours or until the cheese is melted and the edges are browned.

Nutritional Information:

Calories; 295 | Fat: 10 g | Carbohydrates: 16 g | Protein: 24 g

Overnight Oatmeal

Ingredients:
1 liter fat-free milk
1 liter water
340 g steel-cut oats
50 g raisins
75 g dried cherries
65 g dried apricots, chopped
1 teaspoon molasses
1 teaspoon cinnamon (or pumpkin pie spice)

Method:
1. In a slow cooker combine all of the ingredients. Turn heat to low.
2. Put the lid on and cook overnight for 8 to 9 hours.
3. Spoon into bowls and serve.

Nutrition Information:
Calories: 240 | Fat: 3 g | Carbohydrates: 47 g | Protein: 11 g

Sauerkraut Soup

Ingredients:
1 can (about 250 g) of mushroom soup
1 can (about 250 g) of chicken soup
600 ml of water
1 liter of chicken broth
250 g of sauerkraut
1 onion, diced
3 carrots, chopped
5 potatoes, peeled and diced
1 teaspoon of dill weed
1 teaspoon of garlic, minced
½ teaspoon of salt
½ teaspoon of pepper

Method:
1. Peel and dice the potatoes.
2. Cut the carrots and the onions.
3. Mince the garlic.
4. Combine everything into the slow cooker.
5. Put on high heat and cook for four hours.
6. Serve and enjoy.

Nutritional Information:
Calories: 387 | Fat: 23 g | Carbohydrates: 26 g | Protein: 17 g

Sausage with Celery and Chicken

Ingredients:

200 g onions; chopped
100 g celery; chopped
250 ml water
½ teaspoon Cajun season
½ teaspoon thyme dried
500 g skinless chicken (breast or thighs) cut into 1 inch/2 cm cubes
240 g sausage sliced
4 cups cooked rice
450 g canned tomatoes (diced with green chilies) undrained
1 pound medium size shrimp; peeled and deveined
1 kg cooked rice

Method:

1. Combine the first 8 ingredients in slow cooker; cover and cook on low for 6 hours.
2. Stir in shrimp and cook 10 minutes longer on low or until shrimp is done.
3. Serve over hot cooked rice and garnish with chopped green onion if desired.

Nutritional Information:

Calories; 310 | Fat: 9 g | Carbohydrates: 14 g | Protein: 30 g

Cabbage Rolls

Ingredients:

12 large cabbage leaves
450 g onion; chopped
100 g instant rice; uncooked
250 g ground pork; lean
250 g pork breakfast sausage; 50% lean
¼ teaspoon black pepper
450 g can sauerkraut, shredded, drained and rinsed
½ teaspoon caraway seeds
500 ml tomato juice; low sodium
2 tablespoon brown sugar light
3 tablespoons tomato paste

Method:

1. Cook cabbage leaves in boiling water until tender; about 3 to 4 minutes.
2. Sauté onion in skillet for 5 to 7 minutes or until tender; add rice stir and let stand for 15 minutes.
3. Combine rice, pork, and pepper. Fill cabbage leaf with about ¼ of the meat mixture and turn sides in and roll. Repeat for all cabbage leaves.
4. Mix caraway seed with sauerkraut. Put half the sauerkraut mixture into bottom of slow cooker after coating with non-stick spray or cooking oil. Top layer of sauerkraut with half the cabbage rolls. Repeat this step with remaining sauerkraut and cabbage rolls.
5. Combine tomato juice, brown sugar, and tomato paste with a whisk. Pour tomato juice mixture over sauerkraut and cabbage rolls. Cook on low setting for 6 hours and serve.

Nutritional Information:

Calories; 287 | Fat: 11 g | Carbohydrates: 12 g, Protein: 18 g

Sweet and Sour Chicken

Ingredients:
100 g onion; chopped
30 g sugar
75 g ketchup
60 ml orange juice
3 tablespoons corn syrup
3 tablespoons cider vinegar
2 tablespoons soy sauce; low sodium
1 tablespoon grated fresh ginger
500 g skinless chicken, cubed
240 g pineapple chunks
1 bell pepper, large, cut into ¾ inch/1 cm pieces
1 red pepper, large cut into ¾ inch/1 cm pieces
600 g cooked rice

Method:
1. Combine the first 12 ingredients in a slow cooker.
2. Cook on high for 4 hours or 6 hours on low covered.
3. Serve over hot brown rice.

Nutritional Information:
Calories; 332 | Fat: 3 g | Carbohydrates: 7 g | Protein: 18 g

Chickpea Curry

Ingredients:

650 g cauliflower florets, small
400 g peeled and cubed sweet potato
100 g onion; chopped
1 tablespoon curry powder
1 tablespoon brown sugar
1 tablespoon grated ginger, grated
1 ¼ teaspoon salt
2 minced garlic cloves
480 g chickpeas, drained and rinsed
450 g diced tomatoes
400 ml coconut milk, light
1 package (about 450 g) extra-firm tofu, drained
1 tablespoon canola oil
600 g cooked rice
3 tablespoons chopped cilantro, fresh

Method:
1. Combine first 11 ingredients in slow cooker and stir well. Cover and cook on low setting for 5.5 hours or until vegetables are tender.
2. Place tofu on layers of paper towels and cover with additional towels. Press down to absorb excess liquid and cut into ½ inch /1 cm cubes.
3. Heat oil in pan and cook tofu for 8 to 10 minutes or until browned. Stir into mixture in slow cooker.
4. Serve over rice and garnish with cilantro.

Nutritional Information:

Calories; 328 | Fat: 7 g | Carbohydrates: 11 g | Protein: 13 g

Roast Turkey

Ingredients:
200 g onion; chopped
70 g pitted olives
30 g Julienne-cut tomato halves, sun dried
2 tablespoons lemon juice
1½ teaspoon garlic minced
1 teaspoon Greek seasoning mix
½ teaspoon salt
¼ teaspoon pepper
1 trimmed turkey breast, about 2 kg
130 ml fat free chicken broth; low sodium
3 tablespoons all-purpose flour
Thyme sprigs

Method:

1. Put first 9 ingredients in slow cooker. Add half of the chicken broth, cover and cook for 7 hours on low.
2. Whisk the remaining flour and remaining chicken broth and pour into slow cooker. Cook for an additional 30 minutes on low setting.

Nutritional Information:
Calories; 314 | Fat: 5 g | Carbohydrates: 16 g | Protein: 57 g

Potato Soup

Ingredients:
3 slices bacon
100 g onion; chopped
1.5 kg potatoes; peeled and cut into ¼ inch /1 cm thick slices
120 ml water
500 ml chicken broth; low sodium and reduced fat
½ teaspoon salt
½ teaspoon black pepper
500 ml low fat milk
120 g reduced fat cheddar cheese; shredded
120 g sour cream, light
4 teaspoons chopped chives

Method:
1. Cook bacon in skillet until crisp. Remove bacon from pan and add onion to drippings. Sauté for 3 minutes.
2. Put potato slices and onion in slow cooker after coating with non-stick spray. Combine water with the next three ingredients and add to slow cooker. Cover and cook on low heat for 8 hours or until potatoes are tender.
3. Mash mixture with a potato masher. Stir in milk and ¾ cup cheese. Turn heat to high and cook for 20 minutes.
4. Serve in bowls topped with sour cream, chive, and crumbled bacon.

Nutritional Information:
Calories; 259 | Fat: 6 g | Carbohydrates: 9 g | Protein: 13 g

Vegetarian Chili

Ingredients:

450 g can of firm tofu, drained and cubed
460 g canned black beans, drained
450 g canned tomatoes, crushed
600 g onions, chopped
2 red bell peppers, seeded and chopped
2 green bell peppers, seeded and chopped
4 cloves of garlic
2 tsp ground cumin
½ tsp ground black pepper
6 tbsp chili powder
2 tbsp dried oregano
2 tsp salt
2 tbsp white vinegar, distilled
1 tbsp hot pepper sauce
120 ml olive oil, extra virgin

Method:

1. In a large skillet, heat the oil over medium heat.
2. Add the onions to it and cook until softened. Next add in the peppers, tofu and garlic and cook for approximately for ten minutes or until the vegetables start to turn brown and tender.
3. Now cook the beans in a slow cooker over low heat. Stir in all the vegetables and tomatoes and season it.
4. Cover and cook for approximately six to eight hours.

Nutritional Information:

Calories; 445 | Fat: 18 g | Carbohydrates: 58 g | Protein: 21 g

Spinach Sauce Slow Cooker Style

Ingredients:

840 g tomatoes, peeled and crushed
300 g frozen spinach, chopped, thawed and drained
1 onion, chopped
20 g carrot, grated
2 ½ tbsp red pepper, crushed
5 garlic cloves, minced
180 g tomato paste
140 g mushrooms, sliced
2 tbsp dried oregano
2 tbsp salt
2 tbsp dried basil
2 bay leaves
60 ml olive oil, extra virgin

Method:

1. Combine olive oil with spinach, onion, garlic, carrots, tomato paste and mushrooms in a 5 quart/5-6 liter slow cooker.
2. Add in the salt, pepper, oregano, bay leaves and tomatoes.
3. Cover and cook for approximately 4 hours over high heat. After 4 hours are up, stir and reduce the heat to low and cook for an additional 2 hours.

Nutritional Information:

Calories; 176 | Fat: 8 g | Carbohydrates: 25 g | Protein: 7 g

Vegetarian Minestrone

Ingredients:
1.5 liter vegetable broth
450 g kidney beans, drained
840 g tomatoes, crushed
900 g spinach, freshly chopped
1 onion, chopped
2 large carrots, diced
2 celery ribs, diced
1 zucchini
150 g green beans
1 tbsp parsley, minced
3 garlic cloves, minced
¾ tsp thyme, dried
1½ tsp oregano, dried
1 tsp salt
1/3 tsp ground black pepper
50 g elbow macaroni, cooked
25 g Parmesan cheese, finely grated

Method:
1. In a 6 quart/6-7 liter slow cooker, combine the vegetable broth with kidney beans, green beans, tomatoes, onion, zucchini, celery and carrot.
2. Season it with garlic, thyme, parsley, oregano, salt and black pepper.
3. Cook the minestrone on low heat for approximately 7 to 8 hours.
4. Next, stir the spinach and macaroni into the minestrone and allow it to cook for another 15 minutes or so.
5. Top it off with grated Parmesan cheese.

Nutritional Information:
Calories; 138 | Fat: 2 g | Carbohydrates: 25 g | Protein: 7 g

Chickpea-Squash-Lentil-Stew

Ingredients:
150 g of chickpeas
1300 g of squash, peeled and cut into chunks
2 carrots, peeled and sliced
1 onion, chopped
200 g of red lentils
1 liter of vegetable broth
2 tablespoons of tomato paste
1 tablespoon of ginger, minced
1 ½ teaspoons of cumin
1 teaspoon of salt
¼ teaspoon of saffron
¼ teaspoon of pepper
60 ml of lime juice
75 g of peanuts, chopped
20 g of cilantro

Method:
1. Place the beans in a large crock pot and bring to a boil, cook for about an hour.
2. Drain and combine everything but the peanuts and the cilantro in the slow cooker.
3. Cook on low for about five hours.
4. Serve and enjoy, sprinkle with cilantro and peanuts.

Nutritional Information:
Calories: 294 | Fat: 7 g | Carbohydrates: 48 g | Protein: 14 g

Chickpea-Eggplant-Stew

Ingredients:
75 g of mushrooms
750 ml of water
2 eggplants, peeled and cut
3 tablespoons of olive oil
2 onions, sliced
6 cloves of garlic, minced
2 teaspoons of oregano
1 cinnamon stick
1 teaspoon of salt
1 teaspoon of pepper
1 bay leaf
200 g of dried chickpeas
3 tomatoes, chopped
Pinch of parsley

Method:
1. Preheat the oven to 400°F/200°C.
2. Peel and cut the eggplants, cut the mushrooms and everything else that needs to be cut.
3. Place on baking sheet and cook for 6 minutes.
4. Then transfer to the slow cooker.
5. Cook for four hours on high.
6. Remove the cinnamon stick and the bay leaf.
7. Serve and enjoy.

Nutritional Information:
Calories: 219 | Fat: 7 g | Carbohydrates: 33 g | Protein: 9 g

Bean-Barley-Soup

Ingredients:

1 tablespoon of olive oil
1 onion, diced
1 stalk of celery, diced
1 carrot, diced
2.2 liter of water
1 liter of vegetable broth
100 g of pearl barley
60 g of black beans
60 g of great northern beans
60 g of kidney beans
1 tablespoon of chili powder
1 teaspoon of cumin
½ teaspoon of oregano
¾ teaspoon of salt

Method:
1. Cut everything up that needs to be cut and mix it all together in the Dutch oven.
2. Put on low heat and cook for about two and a half hours.
3. Serve and enjoy.

Nutritional Information:
Calories: 205 | Fat: 3 g | Carbohydrates: 35 g | Protein: 11 g

Squash Quinoa Casserole

Ingredients:

360 g of tomatillos, de-husked and chopped
400 g of cherry tomatoes, chopped
1 bell pepper, chopped
50 g of chopped onion
1 tablespoon of lime juice
1 teaspoon of salt
170 g of quinoa
150 g of feta cheese
1 kg of yellow squash, sliced
2 tablespoons of oregano

Method:

1. Chop everything up that needs to get cut.
2. Place everything in the slow cooker and cook on low for four hours.
3. Serve and enjoy.

Nutritional Information:

Calories: 111 | Fat: 3 g | Carbohydrates: 18 g | Protein: 5 g

Imprint

Image sources/Printing information

Pictures cover: depositphotos.com;

@ Zsuriel; @annohoychuk; @zkruger; @ okkijan

ISBN (softcover glossy): 978-3-98500-213-9

IngramSpark – Lightning Source LLC

Mattis Lundqvist

BuchHörnchen-Verlag

Im Schlimm 13

55768 Hoppstädten-Weiersbach (Germany)